Leptin Di Women:

Easy Solution to Get More Energy and Become Healthier

By

Brittany Samons

Table of Contents

Leptin Diet For Women: Easy Solution to Get More Energy and Become Healthier

By Brittany Samons

© Copyright 2014 Brittany Samons

Reproduction or translation of any part of this work beyond that permitted by section 107 or 108 of the 1976 United States Copyright Act without permission of the copyright owner is unlawful. Requests for permission or further information should be addressed to the author.

This publication is designed to provide accurate and authoritative information in regard to the subject matter covered. This work is sold with the understanding that the publisher is not engaged in rendering legal, accounting, or other professional services. If legal advice or other expert assistance is required, the services of a competent professional person should be sought.

First Published, 2014

Printed in the United States of America

Introduction

In accordance with an English maxim 'Don't dig your grave with your personal knife and fork'

Isn't it true that our food is assassinating us by making us heavy, heavier, heaviest?

Moreover, the paradox of the current scenario is that whenever we endeavor to find out the ways and means to increase our metabolism, we are usually provided with deceptive information by the Food Agencies.

Why should that be the situation? (Food for thought eh..!)

Virtually every day, we hear about the widespread plumpness overwhelming the population across the globe and we are given frightful caveats that being flabby amplifies our jeopardy of enduring staid health problems all the way through our lives.

However don't lose heart because there is light at the end of the tunnel!

The best breakthrough having taken place in the current generation is that all across the globe more and more people are becoming sincere about taking the pounds off for good and are much anxious about weight issues in one way or another.

Chapter 1. Factors Responsible for Weight Loss

In spite of all their attempts, some folks are facing failures as far as weight loss is concerned.

What could be the cause?

Though the cause is very straightforward as well as significant yet it is being much overlooked by most of them; when looked at more closely, it has to do with a group of hormones that are known as the weight loss hormones. These chemicals not only control a person's appetite but also direct as to how much weight will be mislaid or acquired.

Influential quantities of these hormones are liberated by the adipose tissue in the body and one of them is Leptin which fastens to the hypothalamus (the hunger control center of the body), to suggest that no more food is required. Whenever you consume a healthy diet, not only the leptin levels become elevated after a meal but also suppression of hunger and burning of calories is initiated. That simply conveys the fact that healthy eating is trouble-free with leptin.

However, that scene changes in case the function of leptin goes wrong e.g. when somebody heretofore holds surplus adipose tissue. In such a case, despite eating a full meal, an individual might feel hungry, thereby causing an additional weight gain.

Leptin in Greek means lean and its purpose is to restrain the craving for food; therefore the deficiency of leptin in the body could lead to an over- indulgence in food and chubbiness. Knowledge of the errand played by this hormone could clarify why some individuals have a yearning for food soon after the intake of a rewarding feast. This hormone not only acts to adjust the ingestion of foodstuff but also plays an important role in the body's ability to burn fat. It does so by sending messages to the hypothalamus-------a small but the most vital part of the brain that manages the thirst and water balance, craving for food and the state of being fed, autonomic regulation, sentiments and sexual desires. The hypothalamus also manages the natural pattern of physiological and behavioral processes that are programmed close to a 24 hour time e.g. sleep-wake cycles, blood pressure, body temperature and the liberation of hormones.

Chapter 2. Features of Leptin

Whenever the matter of hormones is under discussion, it is obvious that women have a better perception of the harm that could be brought about, if the hormones become lopsided. Nevertheless, it is vital that women be coached about everything occurring in their bodies so as to enable them to become well-informed.

Now! Coming back to leptin - also referred to as the Monarch of all hormones (because it keeps an eye on nearly every activity of the hypothalamus of the brain) let's look at the functions being carried out by it:

1.   Adjusts our endocrine system

2.   Fine-tunes our nervous system

3.   Tweaks our metabolism

4.   Lengthens our life

5.   Modifies our energy store-up

When the levels of leptin in the body are well-adjusted, a good number of ailments (such as stoutness, degenerative woes and swelling) are debarred. Leptin not only ascertains how much fat you accrue, but also determines the place where that fat should be accumulated. Whenever people become adamant to leptin, fat gets collected typically around their tummies (apple shaped bodies). This type of obesity puts them at an extensively higher danger of developing diabetes mellitus and heart disease. In case of women, erratic menstrual cycles as well as anxiety is common in such type of obesity. Women who are more liable to build on surplus fat around their bottom (the part of the body that one sits on) hips and thighs (pear shaped bodies) have more prevalence of problems with their blood flow such as varicose veins due to powerful weight around their legs.

Chapter 3. Why It Is Not Easy for Women to Lose Weight?

Again, the fundamental matter of contention is the Leptin hormone. Despite the fact that women possess twofold as much Leptin as men, yet the reaction to Leptin indicators in women is three times smaller than that in men. The malevolent hormone Cortisol compels individuals to stockpile supplementary adipose tissue in their tummies (women being no exception)

In case of women, surplus weight may arrive on the scene due to the inconsistency of the female hormones estrogens and progesterone, which put forward during pregnancy and menopause. Women are more predisposed to stock up more fat than men, because the former develop a reduced basal fat oxidation estimate in contrast to men.

Research scientists accept as true the fact that basal fat oxidation as well as aerobic fitness fall off with age and are decreased in older and overweight women. Moreover, the stuff that may intensify the hazard of escalating obesity comprises serotonin, leptin and insulin; this stuff control women who are likely to attain weight.

Of these, serotonin (a neurotransmitter that serves to adjust the temperature, temperament, violent behavior, frame of mind, annoyance, slumber, sexual drive or interest and appetite)is not only robustly interconnected with the BMI(The body mass index)but is also inversely proportional to it. In case of women, the quantity of serotonin decreases when they achieve a BMI that grades them as plump.

Ghrelin is a hormone that tells your brain to send off more food. Not only it motivates your appetite but also causes tummy flab to build up.

On the other hand, leptin can be thought of as the opposite of ghrelin. When leptin levels are elevated your appetite is scarcely noticeable.

The levels of leptin are higher for girls and women than men at any BMI rank. This is because the female gender has a high adipose tissue mass. Additionally; the quantities of leptin are elevated in women who are heavy with female fetuses as compared to those who are expecting male fetuses. Archetypical diets stimulate the leptin levels of women to nose-dive by reducing the pace and amount on how much they are eating. As a result, they want to eat much even if they are on a diet; this is significant for them to stabilize their hormones, manage appetite and allow their flab to unload. Insulin resistance (which usually takes place secondary to stoutness) also plays a role in bringing about leptin errors. This is because Insulin resistance necessitates more insulin to be employed in order to clean up sugar from the bloodstream. Elevated levels of insulin impede the leptin warning signs (that are making a journey to the brain). As a consequence, your brain supposes that you have a craving for food so that you will be inclined to consume uncalled for calories. This vicious cycle replicates itself so that the hormones become more and more deranged. To compound all this, the hormone ghrelin comes into the picture. This hormone toils between the belly and the hypothalamus. An empty belly causes ghrelin to motivate neurons in the hypothalamus, which inform the brain that it is time to eat. With the intake of food, the tummy widens and another hormone, called cholecystokinin, is liberated.

Now you have an idea that numerous hormones begin to coordinate together to tell the body it is time to discontinue eating. One of the hormones that your body can rely on is peptide YY, which is activated when food tugs into the intestines. So if you disregarded the primary warning sign, you have other depiction to discontinue eating.

When a woman makes an attempt to diet harshly, the leptin levels can go down too much very quickly; as a result, she realizes that it is not very easy to lose weight. In reality, sooner or later, a woman can go through immense back fire gain in weight.

This remarkable escalation and reduction of leptin is the reason for causing so many off-putting diets to be unsuccessful and so many women to acquire all the weight back. This outcome is of poorer quality in women than in men because women have elevated leptin levels to begin with; which deteriorate far lesser than in men when they go on a diet.

Women experience spectacular fluctuations in leptin that necessitate a judiciously designed diet to reduce these considerable fluctuations in leptin levels. One of the practices that have become well-liked is the idea of toting up a dupe day.

Dupe day or cheat day, is a day during the diet program where the women are coached to eat extra food and additional carbohydrates purposely to make an effort to back pedal their leptin levels after days and days of dieting and sinking their leptin levels.

Given that leptin drops faster in women, it is clear that the dupe day or calculated eat-up day is a valuable process for women who should incorporate it all the way through their weight loss agenda; not only this would put off their leptin levels from rolling but would also disallow any bounce back weight gain. Those women who want to keep their leptin levels regular and uniform and also want to burn up their fat, should better add in these calculated eat up days in their weekly plan so that they could get rid of their fat very swiftly.

Chapter 4. Principles and Purposes of Leptin Diet for Women

Leptin diet is the leading manner founded on the discipline of leptin, by which women can watch their waistline. It is a vigorous and chic way of taking care about the categories of food you devour as well as the time when these foods are gulped down. This diet educates women to capitalize on their ability to acquire power from the food they eat In other words even by eating less food they can sense themselves to be outstanding. This regime is very easy and undemanding. Eating in synchronization with leptin rigs out to be the enigma to stimulating the metabolism. Given that the hormone leptin is produced in the fat cells of the body, so when it enters the brain suitably, it grants a metabolic go indicator.

In order to perk up this hormone, the time when a woman eats is as valuable as what she eats.

The five regulations of the leptin diet:

A.   Never ever eat anything subsequent to dinner.

B.   Always eat three meals per day.

C.   Never eat large meals.

D.   Never skip your breakfast; it should categorically comprise protein

E.   Eat carbohydrates only sparingly

Chapter 5. Leptin Resistance

When an individual is chubby, Leptin does not perform very well, on account of his or her brain being unwilling to the appetite-controlling indicators of Leptin. This is known as Leptin resistance or Leptin defiance; it implies that his/her brain believes that the individual is hungry. On the contrary, the actuality is just the reverse. Troubles crop up when a person eats in a style that chokes the entrance of leptin into his/her brain. An example of such a mode of eating is the intake of tidbits (which increase the level of fat found in the blood) during the day; this blocks the ingress of leptin into the brain.

When this occurs, the person acquires a snag known as leptin resistance and the body performs as if it is famished. This establishes massive problems for the body and causes weight gain, swelling and increased risk for many ailments.

The way to dig one's way out of this pothole is to eat in agreement with leptin which is the best dieting approach and the breakdown to do so is the prime reason for global fatness.

Affairs that add to leptin resistance

Leptin resistance is a multifaceted problem with no particular cause; however, there are many issues that can harmfully force Leptin levels:

1.   Consumption of elevated Fructose Corn Syrup

2.   Bigger levels of tension

3.   Utilization of surplus simple carbohydrates such as simple sugars which are processed and have very diminutive dietetic worth to the body.

4.   Deficiency of sleep

5.   Elevated levels of insulin

6.   Disproportionate eating

7.   Too much workout especially if your hormones are already smashed

8.   Consumption of grains and lectin

Chapter 6. How to Repair Leptin Resistance?

Food Recommendations (What to Eat)

1. Eat a healthy nutritious diet comprising 40 percent healthy carbohydrates (such as green vegetables and fruits, whole grains, low-fat dairy products), 30 percent lean protein (such as fish) and 30 percent healthy fats (such as olives, avocadoes, nuts, fatty fish). Consume foods rich in antioxidants (fruits, vegetables, seafood, meat etc) so that the vicious chemicals called Free radicals could be shattered. Eat foods abounding in protein and Omega-3 fatty acids such as cold water fatty fish (e.g. salmon and tuna)scrambled eggs, flaxseeds, hempseeds etc This supports satiation and provides the body the necessary building blocks to make hormones

2. Authorities praise omega-3 fatty acids in salmon with diminishing the levels of leptin. The high protein stuff in fish also assists in cutting back the desire for food, and the advantages of eating the proposed amount reduces a person's risk of being agonized with heart ailment as well as Alzheimer's disease. Salmon contains a notable amount of protein, fatty acids, vitamins and minerals and is amazingly

low in calories; thus it is an ideal serving of food for those who want to uphold a normal weight. Salmon should be integrated in the diet of those persons who are implicated in weight loss plan because it provokes the routine creation and functioning of insulin and puts a stop to insulin resistance, thereby fostering the levels of sugar in the blood; as a result, yearning for food and overeating are prohibited. Patients suffering from DM type 2 gain from this property of omega 3.

3. The Omega 3 from salmon supports the body in blazing calories before they can be piled up and transformed into fats. The Eicosapentaenoic acid - EPA is an omega3fatty acid which motivates the production of Leptin that acts as the body's natural weight management appliance. The Omega 3 fatty acids found in salmon are not only known for their weight loss assets, but also for their ability to protect the heart from certain kinds of ailments. They prevent the arrhythmias, improve the ratio of good cholesterol and act as blood thinners.

4. Spend extravagantly on foods rich in flavonoids and indoles. The former are the phytonutrients found in plant-based food stuffs that often play a role in providing color to the foods e.g. blue berries, cranberries, raspberries, blackberries, red grapes, cherries, plums, citrus fruits

etc.Indoles are found in cauliflower, broccoli, Brussels sprouts, cabbage etc and are beneficial against muscle soreness,pre-menstrual symptoms, menopausal symptoms, malignancies of colon,prostate,ovaries etc

5. Consume dark green leafy vegetables before 10 am by endeavoring to tote up vegetables to your breakfast. In addition to leafy dark green vegetables plenty of fruits should be consumed. The reason for doing so is that vegetables and fruits have excessive nutritional value and high ranking fibers hence they help boost the rate of metabolism. Among the dark green leafy vegetables, spinach is a impressive metabolism booster food because it contains magnesium which assists in smoldering body fat. On account of being jam-packed with nutrients, the body has to struggle more to assimilate them and wheedle out their useful nutrients. Citrus fruits such as grapefruit and oranges possess a high content of vitamin C which also assists in smoldering fat and mounting the rate of metabolism.
Apples and pears are especially counted as weight loss fruits due to their low calorie and rich fiber content.

6. Keep yourself mobile on a regular and constant basis by indulging in some repeated physical activity such as walking

for one hour daily or an exercise such as weight lifting or swimming. This enables the body to blaze flab for energy. However take care not to indulge in any regular exercise if you are leptin resistant; the reason being that if you do so during leptin opposition, you will only add further hassle to the body. It is better to let your body nurse back to health first and then include any workout.

7. Drink plenty of cold filtered water throughout the day. Every so often, that is what the body really needs instead of food.

8. Enhance the ingestion of fiber because fibrous foods are assimilated sluggishly in comparison to the refined foods which hold extra sugar and fat.

9. Endeavor your best to stay away from foods which instigate your insulin levels to be raised. Elevated levels of insulin in the blood mess about with Leptin's communication to the brain. Always select cereals and breads comprising whole grains. The latter are composite carbohydrate foods which possess rich fiber content; they assist in enhancing your metabolism by decelerating the liberation of insulin.

Surplus insulin in the bodily system begins to stockpile foods in the form of fat and decelerates your metabolism.

10. Go out of the rooms barefoot during the day, in noon sun with some skin uncovered.

11. Permit four hours between breakfast and lunch and the same duration between lunch and dinner. Also permit twelve hours amid dinner and breakfast. The idea is to generate suitable phases of burning fat during the day so that the body is facilitated to blaze fat instead of stock piling it.

12. Try to go to sleep by ten pm at night so as to boost your sleep

Food Recommendations (What to Avoid)

1) In keeping with various research studies on the subject of Leptin Resistance, it is apparent that refined carbohydrates such as starches and sugars e.g. high fructose corn syrup and lectins (carbohydrate-binding proteins) which are found in elevated intensity in beans, cereal grains and nuts in the form of additives should be evaded at all costs.

2) Never miss out a meal (in particular breakfast) When you are persistently eating, even little quantities, during the day it carries out continuous working of your liver and doesn't give a rest to the hormones.

3) Do eat three meals each day but taking care to permit a gap of five to six hours between meals.

4) Don't for Heaven's sake eat outsized meals; conclude a meal when you are to some extent fewer than filled.

5) Don't cut out carbohydrates altogether; just restrict them.

6) Don't eat for a minimum of four hours prior to going to bed.

7) Don't drink anything full of calories before going to bed.

8) Reduce the consumption of conventional meats and vegetable oils because they contain Omega-6 fatty acids which enhance the process of inflammation.

9) Never delay your supper or dinner because it is mandatory for you to have a minimal of eleven to twelve hours between dinner and breakfast so as to enable best possible fat burning..

10) Eliminate poisons from your living {as these are a trauma on your body} by getting rid of marketable deodorants and saleable soaps.

11) Avoid doing cardio because it is merely a pressure on the body.

12) Never workout in the mornings; always do so in the evening so as to sustain hormone levels.

Chapter 7. Some Food Recipes for Leptin Diet

1. The revitalizing oatmeal for breakfast

This yummy and comprehensive breakfast recipe is a wonderful way to begin the day. The time for preparation as well as for cooking is not more than ten minutes.

The constituents of the recipe are as follows:

i.   One cup turned over oats

ii.   Two cups water

iii.   Salt according to taste(better use sea salt)

iv.   Half teaspoonfuls cinnamon

v.   Quarter cup raisins

Take water in a saucepan and add sea salt to it. When water and salt simmer, include oats. Heat for about five minutes and take care to swirl frequently so as to sidestep formation of blobs. Put in cinnamon, raisins and almonds; blend and jacket the pan and switch off the heat. Let the mixture lie for five minutes. Dish up with milk and honey. This oatmeal is enough for two persons.

2. The delicious Asian tuna recipe

The preparation time for this recipe is 15 minutes.

Constituents for this recipe are as follows:

i.   Four to six oz tuna steaks

ii.   One tablespoonful fresh lemon juice

iii.   One cup minced spring onions

iv.   Three medium cloves squeezed garlic

v.   One tablespoon pounded fresh ginger

vi.   Two cups densely sliced fresh edible shiitake mushrooms(with detached stems)

vii.   One tablespoon chicken soup

viii.   One cup fresh squeezed orange juice

ix.   Two tablespoonfuls soy sauce

x.   Two tablespoonfuls sliced coriander

xi.   Salt to taste

xii.   White pepper to taste

Method:

Heat the roaster/gas grill on an elevated temperature beforehand and place a stainless steel frying pan about five inches from the heat for around ten minutes to make it scorching. Squeeze garlic and let it be placed for five minutes. Pat tuna with lemon juice and tang with a little salt and white pepper. Keep it in reserve. Heat one tablespoonful soup in a stainless steel roaster on the stove. Cook spring onions, garlic, ginger, and mushrooms in soup for around two minutes, mixing continuously over average heat. Include orange juice and cook for another two minutes. Put in soy sauce and coriander. Using a warm pad, pull out the roaster pan and place tuna in it and restore the saucepan to the roaster. Lay tuna on plates and decant mushroom sauce over each piece. This recipe is enough for four persons.

3. The red kidney bean soup

The process of making this soup ready cum the cooking time add up to thirty-five minutes.

The constituents for the recipe are as follows:

i.   One medium sliced onion

ii.   One medium sliced carrot in pieces of half an inch each

iii.   One stalk celery sliced in pieces of half an inch

iv.   Four medium cloves of sliced garlic

v.   Three cups plus one tablespoon chicken / vegetable soup

vi.   Three tablespoonfuls tomato paste

vii.   One tablespoon crushed cumin

viii.   Two tablespoon red chili powder

ix.   One tablespoon dried oregano

x.   Two cups organic red kidney beans drained

xi.   Salt and pepper to taste

xii.   Half cup plain yogurt

xiii.   One tablespoon lime juice

xiv.   One tablespoon sliced fresh coriander

Method:

Heat up one tablespoonful soup in an average sized soup container. Stir fry onion in soup over medium heat for fifteen minutes; whisk repeatedly until clear. Tote up garlic, carrots, celery and carry on to stir fry for one more minute. Add soup, tomato cream, kidney beans and spices. Let it boil; then decrease heat to medium low and seethe for another fifteen to twenty minutes. Let cool for a few minutes. Prepare lime yogurt by blending yogurt, lime juice, and coriander in discrete little bowl. Mix the soup on a low speed blender. Tang with salt and pepper to taste. Before serving, do heat it again and shift into serving bowls; Crown with a spoonful of lime yogurt, and dish up. The recipe is enough for four persons.

Conclusion

The satiety hormone Leptin is the concierge of fat metabolism which supervises the amount of energy an individual captures. Not only it evaluates and upholds the energy balance in the body, but also adjusts appetite. In order to increase your production of leptin, eat foods which are rich in protein, zinc (oysters, redmeat and whole grains are good sources of zinc) and omega-3 fatty acids.

Lofty levels of leptin have been associated with hypertension, corpulence, heart ailment and stroke, as well as troubles associated with blood sugar.

Elevated levels of Leptin and the associated leptin opposition can also reduce productiveness, let you grow old more hastily and have a say in stoutness. Leptin is created by fat cells, so it would appear reasonable that those with more plump cells would produce extra Leptin, which would signify the body to eat a lesser amount of food and weight would standardize.

The bottom line

The bottom line is that vigorous leptin operation is linked with mainstay endurance and proper health. Eating in agreement with leptin is for all and sundry at every body weight. The inability to eat in synchronization with leptin is the primary reason for the global obesity.

Thank You Page

I want to personally thank you for reading my book. I hope you found information in this book useful and I would be very grateful if you could leave your honest review about this book. I certainly want to thank you in advance for doing this.

Lightning Source UK Ltd.
Milton Keynes UK
UKOW06f0636070415

249226UK00010B/215/P

9 781633 832671